I0765668

# TABLE OF CONTENTS

## INTRODUCTION

The role of keto within the treatment of wellness has been best-known to the human race for thousands of years and was studied thoroughly by Greek physicians and ancient Indian physicians. An early piece of writing within the medical practitioner Corpus, "On the Sacred wellness," describes the needs of keto. However, alterations in diet contend a task in health management. A similar author additionally describes in "Epidemics" from the gathering, yet a person was cured of health once he abstained fully from overwhelming food or drink.

## HISTORY OF KETO DIET

The ketogenic diet became in style as a medical care for health within the 20s and 30s. It developed to produce an alternate to non-mainstream abstinence that had success as health medical care. However, the diet was eventually mostly abandoned because of the introduction of the latest antiepileptic drug therapies. Though it emerged that almost all cases of encephalopathy might effectively control the exploitation of these medications, they still did not deliver the goods epileptic management in around two hundredths to a half-hour of people with epilepsy. For these people, and notably kids with encephalopathy, the diet re-introduced as a way of managing the condition.

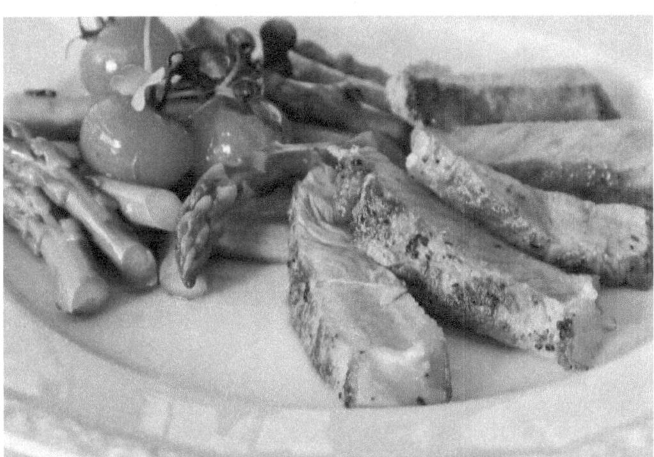

In 1911, the first scientific study into abstinence as a cure for encephalopathy conducted in France. At the time, the restrainer was accustomed to treat people with epilepsy. However, this agent slowed patients' mental capabilities. Instead, twenty encephalopathy patients followed a low-calorie, feeder food set up that was combined with abstinence. 2 patients showed vital enhancements, though most couldn't adhere to the dietary restrictions. However, the diet was found to enhance the patient's mental skills compared with the consequences of taking restrainer.

## KETO DIET ON THIS CENTURY

Also, throughout the first twentieth Century, a yank referred to as Bernarr Macfadden, popularized the thought of abstinence as a way of restoring health. His student therapist, Hugh Conklin, introduced abstinence as a treatment technique for dominant health. Colin projected that epileptic seizures caused by a poisonous substance secreted within the viscous and instructed that abstinence for eighteen to twenty-five days may cause the toxic substance to dissipate. His epileptic patients were placed on a "water diet," that he, according to cured ninetieth of youngsters with the condition and five-hundredths of adults.

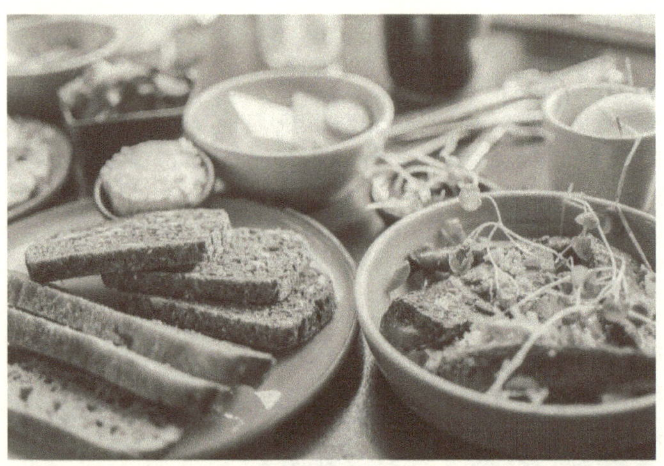

Analysis of the study that performed later showed that two-hundredths of Conklin's patients became seizure-free, whereas five-hundredths incontestable some improvement. The abstinence medical care shortly adopted as a part of thought medical care for encephalopathy. Moreover, in 1916, Dr. McMurray, according to the big apple Medical Journal that he had with success, treated epileptic patients by prescribing a quick, followed by a diet freed from starch and sugar since 1912.

It was in 1921 that medical specialist Rollin Woodyatt noted that the liver created three soluble compounds, acetone, β-hydroxybutyrate, and acetoacetate as a result of starvation or if they followed a diet made in fat and low in carbohydrates. In 1921, Russel Wilder from the mayonnaise Clinic referred to this as the "ketogenic diet" and used it as a treatment for encephalopathy.

Further analysis within the Sixties showed that additional ketones area unit created by medium-chain triglycerides per unit of energy as a result of their transported quickly to the liver as critical the system lymphatic. In 1971, Peter Huttenlocher devised a ketogenic diet where calories came from MCT oil that allowed new macromolecule and carbohydrates to be enclosed. Compared with the initial ketogenic diet, it means folks may prepare additional meals for his or her youngsters with health.

## WHAT IS KETOGENIC DIET

This diet is termed ketogenic as a result of it mimics the consequences of fast that causes the body to provide ketones. Throughout starvation, the body is forced to burn fats instead of carbohydrates. During a ketogenic diet, the most supply of energy is fat, and once this often combined with the occasional intake of carbohydrates, the body makes ketones.

The brain sometimes depends on aldohexose as energy supply; however, once insufficient carbohydrates are offered; the liver processes fats to supply the brain with energy within the type of fatty acids and organic compound bodies. The hyperbolic blood level of natural compound bodies is brought up as acetonemia. The ketogenic diet is related to seizure reduction in youngsters with a brain disease that's troublesome to manage.

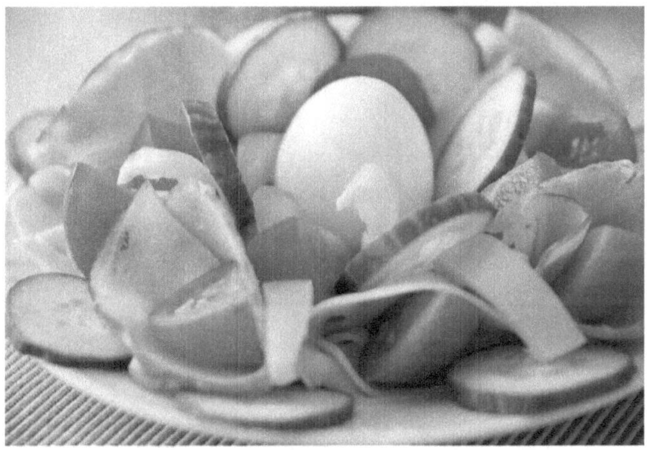

The ketogenic diet contains an amount of supermolecule for body growth and repair. The overall calories within the food are also comfortable to keep up a healthy weight for a given age and height.

In the classic ketogenic diet, the quantitative relation of fats to carbohydrates and proteins combined is 4:1. Samples of the high-fat foods eaten embrace butter, cream, lard, oil, and duck fat and examples of high-carbohydrate foods to avoid embrace grains, bread, pasta, sugar, starchy fruits.

**WHAT IS KETONE**

From fat, your diet into molecules referred to as ketones, another supply of fuel. It puts you into ketonemia, aka prime weight loss mode. In keto once, your organic compound levels live 0.8 millimoles per liter. The keto diet is a technique to urge your body to form ketones. Different ways in which to run on ketones embrace intermittent fast and consumption your aldohexose reserves by physical exertion.

The keto diet quickly boosts weight loss as a result of your body turns fat from your food and your fat stores into ketones. Moreover, in contrast to aldohexose, ketones can't be kept as fat. As a result of they aren't digestible identical means. For many years, you've detected that fat causes you to fat. Your body is designed to use fat as another supply of fuel. For many of history, individuals weren't uptake three meals and snacks throughout the day. Instead, humans would get to hunt and gather their food, and that they learned to thrive once there wasn't any food on the market, typically for days on finish. Their bodies used to keep fat for energy.

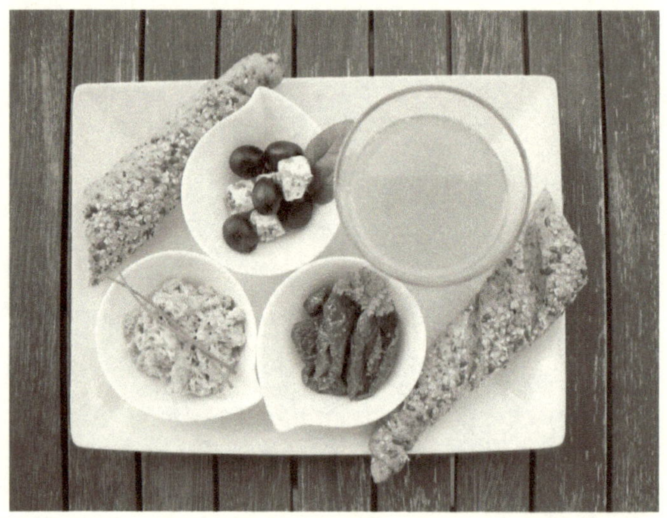

**MANY EDGES OF A KETOGENIC DIET**
**Burns Body Fat**

Once you're on keto, your body uses keep body fat and fat from your diet as fuel. Get a speedy weight loss.

**Reduces Appetite**

Ketone suppresses endocrine and uses to decrease hunger. Increase cholecystokinin, which causes you to feel full. Reduced appetence means that it's easier to travel for extended periods while no uptake, which inspires your body to read its fat stores for energy.

## Reduces Inflammation

Inflammation is your body's natural response to intruder it deems harmful. An excessive amount of swelling is unhealthy news as a result of it will increase your risk of chronic wellness. A keto diet will scale back inflammation within the body by switch off inflammatory pathways and manufacturing fewer free radicals compared to aldohexose.

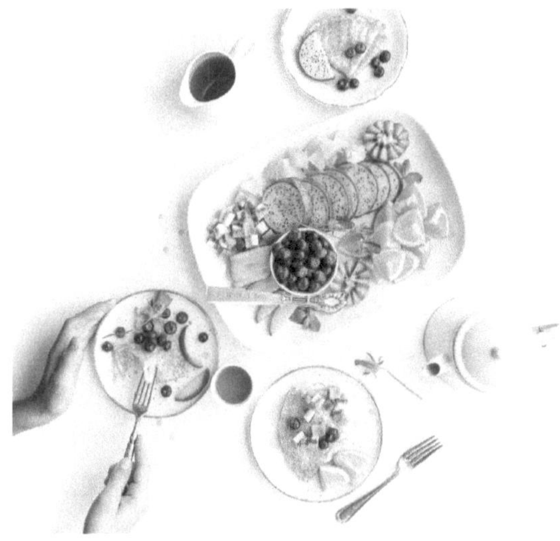

## Fuels Your Brain

It wants, that is far a lot of economical than the power you get from aldohexose. You recognize your mind created of over sixty percent fat. Meaning it wants heaps of fat to stay the engine buzzing. The high fats you vex a ketogenic diet do overfeed your daily activities — they conjointly feed your brain.

## Increases Energy

Once your brain uses ketones for fuel, you are doing expertise identical energy slumps. You do once you're uptake heaps of carbs. Once your metabolism is in fat-burning mode, your body will use merely faucet into it without delay on the market. The fat stores for energy mean any energy crashes. Ketonemia conjointly helps the brain produce many mitochondria, the ability generators in your cells. Much energy in your cells means that much power to urge stuff done.

## Curbs Cravings

Fat may be a super satiating macronutrient. You eat a lot of high fats on keto. Therefore you're feeling fuller, longer.

## TYPES OF KETO DIETS

**Standard keto:** You eat low carb, every day. Some keto followers eat as few as twenty grams per day.

**Cyclical keto:** Eat a high-fat, terribly low-carb 5 to 6 days per week. On day seven, have a carb reefed day. The Bulletproof Diet falls into this class. However, tweaks keto for even higher performance with periodic abstinence, macromolecule abstinence, and stress on nutrient-dense, low-inflammation foods. Transfer the Bulletproof Diet Roadmap at no cost here.

**Targeted keto:** You follow the quality keto diet; however, eat additional carbs half-hour to an hour before a high-intensity sweat. The aldohexose is supposed to spice up performance. Moreover, you come to acetonemia when sweat. If your energy is suffering within the gymnasium throughout keto, this variety of intake may work for you.

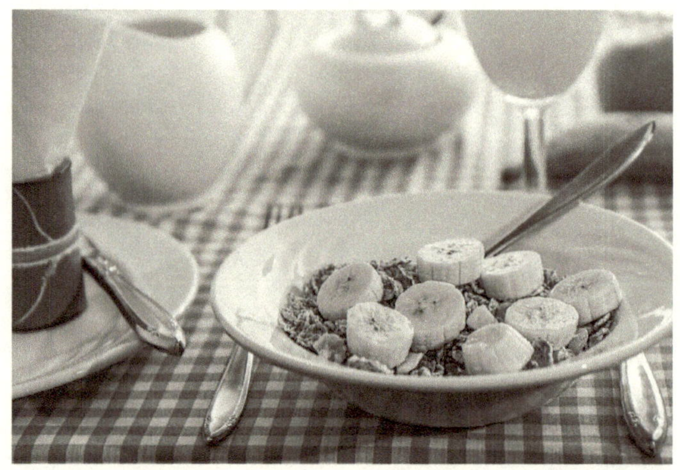

**Dirty keto:** Dirty keto follows an equivalent quantitative relation of fats, proteins, and carbs because of the regular keto diet. However, with a twist, it doesn't matter wherever those macronutrients return. Dinner might be massive bundles with a Diet Pepsi Cola. Learn much concerning the dirty keto diet and the way it works.

**Moderate keto:** Eat high fat with 100-150 grams of web carbs daily. Ladies usually do best with this diet limiting carbs will typically mess with secretion operates. Also, some athletes realize they break with fewer than one hundred grams of carbs on sweat days.

## BENEFITS OF VEGETABLES ON KETO DIET

Vegetables are healthy and alimentary foods. Plants offer energy, vitamins, minerals, and fiber, and there's growing proof of extra health advantages from a variety of phytonutrients. Some vegetables contain higher levels of the supermolecule and are, typically known as starchy vegetables. These are usually roots and tubers like potatoes, yams, kumara, taro, and sweet corn. The greens are higher in energy thanks to their supermolecule content. Other vegetables classified as non-starchy. Non-starchy plants tend to own the following water content, and are lower in energy; however typically richer in vitamins and minerals.

## 1. KALE

A more fat-soluble vitamin that is sweet for your blood and carotenoid good for your eyes than you would like for the day. Moreover, many antioxidants smart for your system, heart, skin, and plenty of alternative stuff too. Glucosinolates in kale could scale back the chance of sure kinds of cancer by boosting enzymes.

## 2. SPINACH

Spinach meets your daily necessities for fat-soluble vitamin and carotenoid and has many antioxidants and atomic number 19 smart for your muscles and heart too. It even throws in some fiber smart for pooping live.

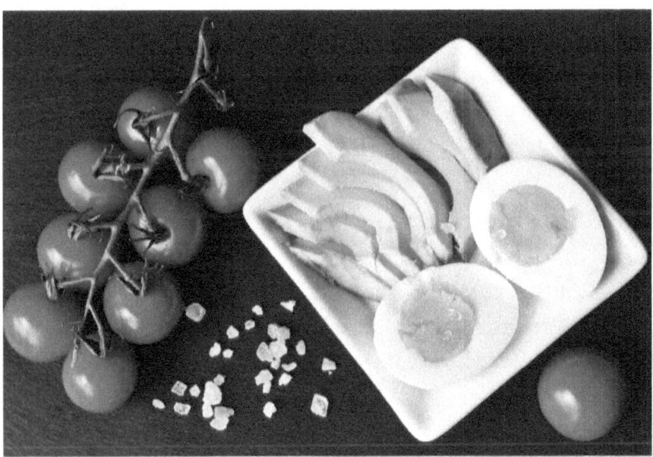

## 3. CARROTS

Falcarinol in carrot has attracted interest for his or her potential as anti-cancer compounds. However, at high levels, these compounds may be toxic.

## 4. TOMATOES

With that entire antiophthalmic factor boosts your immunity, vision, and fruitful health. Moreover, C, you ought to in all probability toast yourself for having some. Over the past decade, scientists became more and more curious about the potential for numerous dietary flavonoids to elucidate a number of the health advantages related to fruit- and vegetable-rich diets. Health advantages embody reducing cancer, polygenic disorder, and heart condition risk, serving to maintain healthy bones, brain, and vision.

## 5. BEETROOT

The battalions in beetroots have received less attention than the additional standard natural red pigments, the anthocyanin. However, analysis indicates they need medicine properties and will boost the body's detoxification enzymes.

## BENEFITS OF FRUITS ON KETO DIET

Fruits don't seem to be solely delicious, however healthful too. Made in vitamins A and C, and folic acid and different essential nutrients, they will facilitate forestall cardiopathy and stroke, management pressure and steroid alcohol, forestall some forms of cancer and guard against vision loss. They are therefore smart for you that Health North American country recommends that almost all girls get servings of fruit and vegetables daily. If it is the vitamins that promote healthiness, you will marvel if you'll pop supplements. Nope. Covered peaches and vine-ripened grapes contain quite only vitamins. They are an excellent combination of fiber, minerals, antioxidants, and phytochemicals, yet because of the vitamins that employment together to produce protecting advantages.

## 1. LEMONS

Lemons are an edible fruit that individuals typically use in ancient remedies as a result of their health advantages. Like different citrus fruits, they contain vitamin C and various antioxidants. Antioxidants square measure essential for human health. These compounds mop up free radicals within the body that may harm the body's cells and cause diseases, like cancers.

## 2. STRAWBERRIES

Strawberries are a juicy, red fruit with high water content. The seeds give lots of dietary fiber per serving. Berries contain several healthful vitamins and minerals. Of explicit note, they contain anthocyanin that is flavonoids that may facilitate boost heart health. The fiber and atomic number 19 in strawberries may also support a healthy heart.

## 3. ORANGES

Oranges are a sweet, spherical edible fruit filled with vitamins and minerals. Oranges square measure among the richest sources of vitamin C, with one medium fruit providing 117 % of a daily human price of vitamin C.

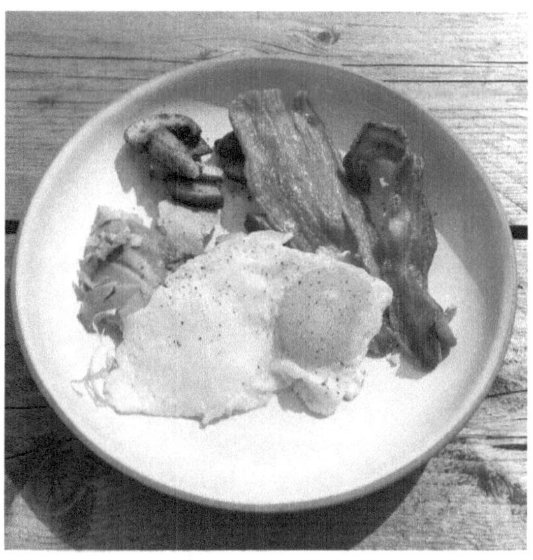

## 4. APPLES

Apples build a fast and straightforward addition to the diet. Eat them with the skin on for the best health advantages. Apples are high-fiber fruits that mean that feeding them may boost heart health and promote weight loss. The cellulose in apples helps to keep up sensible gut health.

## 5. BANANAS

Bananas square measure documented for his or her high atomic number 19 content. A medium banana contains 422 mg of the adequate adult intake of 4,500 mg of atomic number 19. It helps the body management pulse and pressure level. Bananas are an honest supply of energy, with one banana containing a hundred and five calories and twenty 6.95 g of the supermolecule. The 3.1 g of fiber during a regular banana may also facilitate with regular viscous movements and abdomen problems, like ulcers and redness.


**TOP FIFTEEN DETOX JUICE RECIPES FOR KETO DIET**

Here are a number of the foremost standard juice recipes, for we have a tendency to weight loss we found to grant you some concepts for a do-it-yourself juice cleanse. Perpetually be happy to experiment with new ingredients, and you'll never be uninterested in detox juice.

Always use organic ingredients whenever doable to scale back the danger of poisons. Every formula makes two servings.

## 1. THE GREEN DETOX JUICE

This delicious detox juice formula is one in all the foremost standard recipes offered. It's the right balance of fruits and vegetables. It makes an ideal mix for detoxing your body when the vacations or a celebration.

Apple is choked with nutrition. Additionally, to being a decent supply of antioxidants, apples additionally contain polyphenols, which might have various health advantages.

Add or compute the apple servings to form it additional or less sweet in step with your style.

### INGREDIENTS

- Two apples cut in half
- Three stalks celery, no leaves
- One cucumber
- Eight leaves kale
- 1/2 lemon, peeled
- One-piece contemporary ginger
- A spring of mint

Once you prepared, merely method all the ingredients along in your favorite liquidizer, shake or stir, then serve.


## 2. HEALTHY CARROT APPLE JUICE

It is an incredibly delicious drink and choked with helpful nutrients like vitamins, minerals, and antioxidants.

Carrots are an excellent supply of vitamin A within the style of beta carotene. They're conjointly a superb supply of B vitamins, vitamin K and K.

The juice is pleasantly sweet, and pairs well with the tartness of the apples. Once shopping for apples, opt for firm ones as they're going to manufacture a more transparent juice.

### INGREDIENTS

- One massive apple quartered
- 1/4 (15 ounces) will pineapple chunks
- Two enormous carrots
- Two items ginger

Throw every one of these things into your liquidizer, alongside your washed kale and celery, and Blitz till swish. Pour into glasses and garnish as your choice.

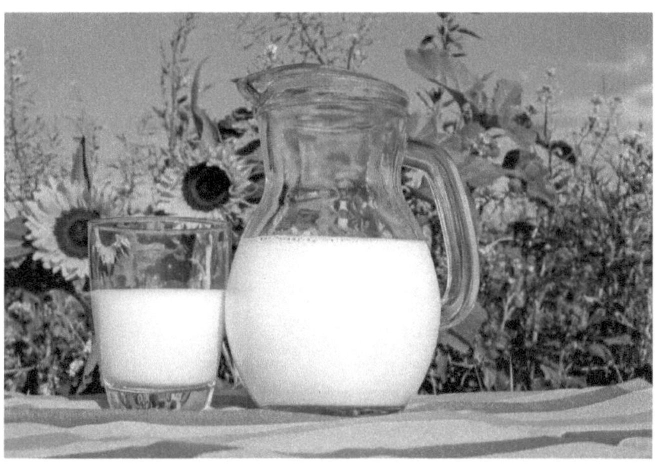

## 3. ZESTY LEMON DETOX

It is an amazingly lightweight and tart drink that creates an ideal juice for breakfast or early within the morning.

Besides all the antioxidants within the apples and lemons, the cucumbers have several health edges also, together with vitamin K.

### INGREDIENTS

- Two lemons, raw and halved
- Four apples, quartered
- Two cucumbers halved
- 1 cup of water

Mix them all in the blender machine and serve.


## 4. CHILD-FRIENDLY DETOX JUICE

If you're searching for juice direction for youths they're going to love, this can be an honest one. The fruits do a reasonable job of masking the style of the vegetables, and this direction tastes specialized.

Spinach is an excellent supply of many vitamins and minerals. It contains high amounts of carotenoids, vitamin C, vitamin K, folic acid, iron, and atomic number 20.

**INGREDIENTS**

- Two oranges, peeled
- One lemon, peeled
- One apple quartered
- 1 cup spinach
- One leaf kale

Once you prepared, merely method all the ingredients along in your favorite liquidizer, shake or stir, then serve.


## 5. RED DETOX BREAKFAST JUICE

Here's another excellent juice ward to begin your morning. It's got a unique nutrition profile from the vegetables and fruits, and it tastes sweet, with a small kick from the lemons.

The beets are an honest supply of vitamins and minerals, like Focalin, potassium, manganese, iron, and water-soluble vitamin.

**INGREDIENTS**

- Two lemons
- Two carrots
- Two apples
- Two beets

Throw every one of these things into your liquidizer, alongside your washed kale and celery, and Blitz till swish. Pour into glasses and garnish as you choose.


## 6. SPINACH FRUIT DRINK

This typical detox drink provides you a lot of energy, and is admittedly smart for you, too. You will need to feature touch honey if you wish it sweeter. Kale is admittedly high in nutrients and low in calories that make it one in all the foremost nutrient-dense foods obtainable.

**INGREDIENTS**

- 1 cup spinach
- Two stalks celery
- Four leaves kale
- One piece of ginger

- Two apples
- One lemon

Mix them all in the blender machine and serve.


## 7. ALLERGIC REACTION FIGHTING JUICE

If you suffer from seasonal allergies, you ought to do that proper health juice instruction. It's allergic reaction fighting ascorbic acid-rich fruits and vegetables like pineapple, lemon, and grapes. Parsley could be a smart supply of fat-soluble vitamin and ascorbic acid, likewise as a fat-soluble vitamin, Focalin, and iron.

### INGREDIENTS

- One cucumber
- 1 cup pineapple
- One lemon
- 1 cup stone fewer grapes
- 1/2 cup parsley
- One apple
- 1 Ming dynasty sprig (optional)

Throw every one of these things into your liquidizer, alongside your washed kale and celery, and Blitz till swish. Pour into glasses and garnish as you choose.


## 8. ORANGE DETOX JUICE

This juice is creamy and delicious, a bit like the previous Orange frozen dessert bars you bear in mind ingestion once you were a child. You'll even freeze these in ice molds for an excellent frozen treat. Pears are a decent supply of many essential nutrients, like fat-soluble vitamin, vitamin C, copper, and metallic element.

### INGREDIENTS

- Two medium apples
- Three stalks celery
- One orange (peeled)
- Two medium pears
- One sweet potato

Make a mixture of the ingredients using a blender machine and serve.

## 9. SIMPLE BEGIN DETOX JUICE

It makes a decent beginner detox juice direction for those only beginning out with juicing because of its straightforward ingredients and delicious flavors that aren't overwhelming.

Carrots have tons of health advantages. They're a decent ingredient once juicing for weight loss and joined to lower cholesterol levels and improved eye health.

**INGREDIENTS**

- Two medium apples
- Three medium carrots
- Four celery stalks

Throw every one of these things into your liquidizer, alongside your washed kale and celery, and Blitz till swish. Pour into glasses and garnish as you choose.

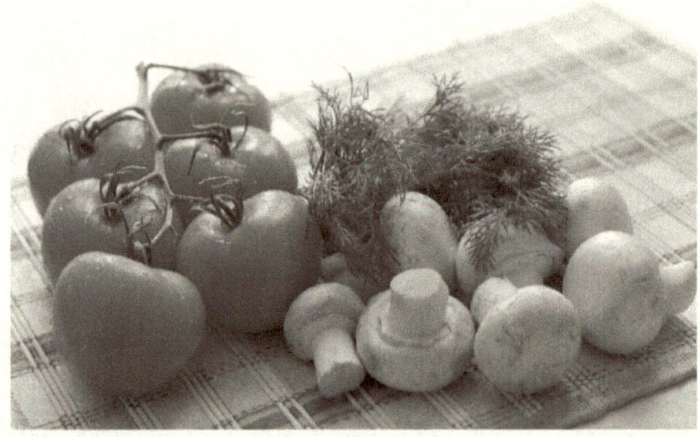

## 10. GREEN GINGER POP

It is my head to direction, particularly once I'm having tummy problems. The style is superb, and it's jam-packed with nutrients because of the variability of ingredients.

Ginger could be a wondrous spice. Only one – 1/2 grams of ginger will facilitate stop varied varieties of nausea like ocean illness, therapy nausea, nausea once surgery, and sickness.

**INGREDIENTS**

- Three medium apples

- Two stalks celery
- 1 cup spinach
- One cucumber
- One piece of ginger root
- One lime (peeled)

Once you prepared, merely method all the ingredients along in your favorite liquidizer, shake or stir, then serve.


## 11. BEETS AND TREATS

The Beets and Treats detox is wealthy in beet juice that helps to clear digestive juice and cleanse away toxicity of blood and liver. The healthier your liver is, the additional it will metabolize fat for fast, natural weight loss.

### INGREDIENTS

- Beetroot (1 beet)
- Two leaves of cabbage (red)
- Three medium carrots
- 1/2 a fruiting lemon
- One whole orange
- 1/4 a fruit pineapple
- One handful spinach

Once you prepared, merely method all the ingredients along in your favorite liquidizer, shake or stir, then serve.


## 12. GREEN AID

Start a great digestion system that it has to begin burning away excess fat with a fast and refreshing juice that you will drink all day long. The more straightforward it's for your body to interrupt down the nutrients and minerals in your food, the less probably you're to struggle with bloating and constipation.

### INGREDIENTS

- Four medium apples
- Three stalks of celery
- Two leaves of kale

- One whole lemon
- 4 cups of spinach

To make this juice, begin by chopping your apples, celery, and lemon into chunks. Throw every one of these things into your liquidizer, alongside your washed kale and celery, and Blitz till swish. Pour into glasses and garnish as you choose.


## 13. ANY TIME FAT LOSS JUICE

Some homemade juice recipes for weight loss square measure good for the morning - once you are still blear from the bed. Alternative methods square measure the proper thanks to wind down when a protracted day at work. The "Any-Time Fat-Loss" cocktail is one amongst those unique blends that job utterly in spite of after you drink it.

## INGREDIENTS

- Two medium apples
- Two stalks of celery
- One whole cucumber
- Five leaves of kale
- 1/2 fruit lemon
- Two whole oranges
- parsley

Chop the parsley and kale along, and then dice the apple, cucumber, celery, lemon, and oranges into chunks. Pour the complete ingredient combine into a liquidizer and Blitz till swish. Stir, pour into a glass and garnish.


## 14. FRUIT DRINK BLITZ

The Green fruit drink Blitz combines the fat-burning power of lemon with the complexion-boosting radiance of cucumber. In alternative words, - you will not solely turn. However, your skin is going to be glowing too.

## INGREDIENTS

- 2 cups of spinach
- One whole lemon
- Four leaves of kale
- One whole cucumber

- Two medium apples

Mix apples and cucumber into manageable chunks and throw them into your juicer, besides your lemon, spinach, and kale. Blitz the complete mixture till swish, and serve during a tall glass with many cubes of ice.


## 15. WINGMAN

The celery and orange in your "Wingman" mix can facilitate to take care of a young sonority in your skin because of a healthy dose of antioxidant, whereas the juice at the same time battles to burn away fat and cure skin-problems with its inherent antiseptic properties.

### INGREDIENTS

- Three whole apples
- Three stalks of celery
- 1/2 vegetable cucumber
- 1/2 thumb of ginger root
- Four leaves of kale
- One whole lemon
- One whole significant orange

Dice the celery, cucumber, lemon, apples, and ginger root into chunks, and throw them into your juices. Add the kale, and blitz the complete mixture till swish. Serve cold.


## TOP FIFTEEN HEALTHY SMOOTHIE RECIPES FOR KETO DIET

Sometimes, attempting to come back up with totally different variations and combos of fruits and vegetables in smoothies and juices will get overwhelming. Thus this assortment of smoothie and juice recipes is meant to create it a no brainer. Of course, be happy to swap in and swap out your favorite ingredients, or modify these recipes supported what you've got on the market.

Here are fifteen awesome and healthy smoothie recipes for you to start your healthy life.

## 1. DAIRY-FREE MANGO COCONUT MILK SMOOTHIE

When you're probing chemo, keeping your weight up may be a challenge, particularly if your appetency is waning. Then it's the most straightforward smoothie for you.

### INGREDIENTS

- One mango or one cup of froze mango chunks
- 1/2 cup fruit crush

- 1/4 cup coconut milk
- One wedge juice squeezed
- One tablespoon flaxseed oil
- One tablespoon copra oil
- 1-2 teaspoons honey to style
- 1/2 cup non-dairy milk I used cashew milk
- Fresh mint leaves for garnish, optional

Put all ingredients during a robust liquidizer and mix it till sleek. For a frostier texture, add some ice cubes.

## 2. BANANA OAT CHOCOLATE SPREAD SMOOTHIE

This smoothie is full of goodness supermolecule from Silk organic soy milk, spread, and oats, K from the bananas, and deliciously wealthy cocoa. You'll get forty-fifths of your Calcium daily demand and 13.5 grams of a supermolecule from a glass of this smoothie within the morning. Moreover, as a result of all the ingredients is plant-based, there's no cholesterol.

**INGREDIENTS**

- 1 cup Silk Vanilla Soy Milk
- 1/2 cup frozen banana slices
- Two tablespoons oats
- One tablespoon spread or alternative seed butter
- One teaspoon non-sweet cocoa

Place all ingredients during a liquidizer and mix it till swish.

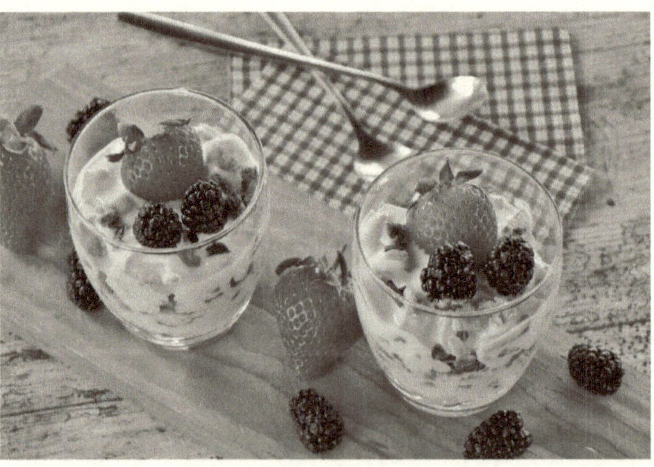

# 3. BANANA KALE SMOOTHIE

Drinking this smoothie was like giving me associate degree infusion of nutrition quickly. It gave a burst of energy before my effort.

## INGREDIENTS

- One pack is frozen acai, broken into chunks
- 1 cup kale leaves loosely packed
- One medium banana
- 1/2 cup organic low-fat vanilla yogurt
- 1/2 cup low-fat organic milk

Place all ingredients during a mixer and mix it till sleek.


# 4. STRAWBERRY AND GREEN TEA SMOOTHIE

This smoothie has one serving of fruit together with chia seeds that area unit wealthy in omega-3 fatty acid fatty acids, protein, fiber, antioxidants, and atomic number 20. Additionally, I added a teaspoon of tea leaf, that is ground, steamed tea leaf leaves, and contains a potent level of antioxidants.

## INGREDIENTS

- 1/2 cup fruit juice
- One tablespoon chia seeds
- 1/2 cup strawberries
- One teaspoon tea leaf powder
- Ice cubes if desired

Soak chia seeds in fruit juice for quarter-hour. Place all ingredients in a liquidizer and mix it till sleek. Use some ice if you prefer a thicker colder smoothie.


# 5. BLUEBERRY BANANA SMOOTHIE

Use your favorite fruit. If you utilize contemporary fruit rather than frozen fruit, merely cut back the quantity of fruit juice and add some ice cubes.

## INGREDIENTS

- 1/2 cup frozen blueberries

- 1/2 cup frozen banana slices or one medium banana troubler
- 1/2 cup non-fat Greek Food
- 1/2 cup fruit juice

Place all ingredients in a liquidizer. Mix till swish.

## 6. FRUITS AND GREEN TEA SMOOTHIE

This formula uses additional fruits than vegetables. Therefore though this smoothie undoubtedly experienced, it tastes fruity, not vegetal.

### INGREDIENTS

- One one/2 cups inexperienced grapes
- 1 cup baby spinach
- 1 cup frozen banana slices
- 1 cup of tea leaf coffee for teenagers

Put all parts in an exceeding liquidizer and mix till swish.

## 7. DETOX BEET AND CARROT SMOOTHIE

It's all the health advantages of 2 superfood vegetables – carrots and beets. Every one of the ingredients during this smoothie has distinctive and powerful antioxidants that facilitate detoxify our bodies and destroy free radicals that work disturbance on our systems.

### INGREDIENTS

- One carrot raw, sliced
- One beet fresh, sliced
- 1/2 cup red grapes
- One clementine raw
- One slice of ginger cold, concerning the scale of 1 / 4
- 1/2 cup tea leaf

Steam carrot and beet till naturally tender, concerning 10-15 minutes, reckoning on, however, thick your slices. Let cool. Place all ingredients in a liquidizer and mix it till swish.

## 8. PEACH AND GREEN TEA SMOOTHIE

If you prefer to drink green tea daily, then you're in all probability to the very fact that green tea has many health edges. It is understood to treat headaches and upset stomach and conjointly acts as a potent inhibitor likewise. Not solely that, however, it may also facilitate fight bacterium and infections, increase weight loss, and probably even stop some varieties of cancer.

**INGREDIENTS**

- One peach
- ½ a banana
- One tea leaf bag
- ½ cup of ice cubes
- One tablespoon of honey

Brew ½ cup of green tea and so chill the tea with ice cubes or place it within the white goods. Then you mix the green tea, banana, and peach during a liquidizer till it's sleek, and add some honey for sweetness.


## 9. GREEN TEA AND ALMOND SMOOTHIE

By adding almonds to your green tea smoothie, it'll not solely offer your smoothie with a bit of many flavors. However, conjointly provides it an additional supermolecule likewise. Also, together with the dairy product in your smoothie, it'll facilitate your gastrointestinal system. The dairy product is understood to fight any bacterium that's in your abdomen.

**INGREDIENTS**

- ¼ cup of sliced almonds
- Four tablespoons of honey
- 1 cup of green tea
- ½ cup of plain or vanilla dairy product

First, mix all the almonds and, therefore, the one tablespoon of honey into the liquidizer, and blend on high speed for regarding 2 to a few minutes till the mixture is sleek. Then add the green tea, yogurt, and, therefore, the remainder of the honey and mix it. However, confirm you mix the honey incorrectly before you add any ice.


## 10. HEALTHY HEALING FRUIT SMOOTHIE

Chia seeds are surprisingly high in fiber and atomic number 20 and are wealthy in polyunsaturated fatty acid fatty acids. They're dull to include in everyday meals. Some individuals prefer to sprinkle Chia seeds on their breakfast cereal.

## INGREDIENTS

- One tablespoon chia seeds
- Two tablespoons water
- One tablespoon contemporary aloe juice
- 1 cup frozen fruit of your selection
- 1 cup almond or different nut milk
- Two tablespoons lightweight coconut milk optional

Soak chia seeds in water for quarter-hour. Place in liquidizer along with side aloe juice, fruit, almond milk, and coconut milk. Mix till swish.


## 11. MANGO COCONUT MINT SMOOTHIE

It'll be necessary to pack a supermolecule and nutrition into each sip or bite. This smoothie direction uses Greek yogurt that is incredibly high in a supermolecule.

## INGREDIENTS

- Two mangoes flesh solely
- 1 cup vanilla non-fat Greek yogurt
- 1 cup milk
- 1/4 cup coconut milk
- A few mint leaves regarding one tablespoon

Place all ingredients in a very liquidizer and mix it till swish. Add much milk if a dilatant consistency desired.

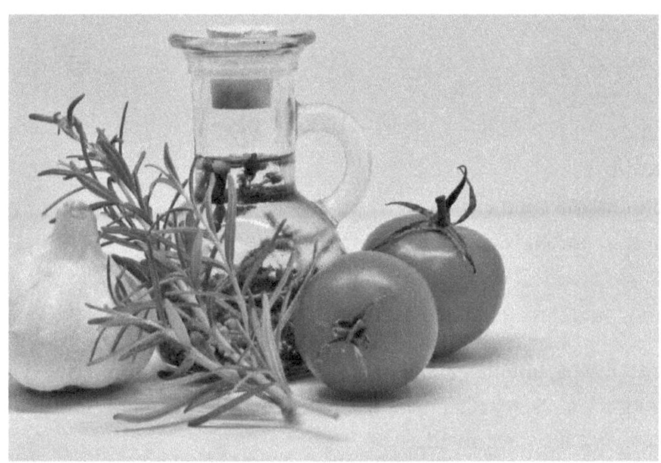

## 12. GUAVA PINEAPPLE BANANA SMOOTHIE

Guavas have a sweet exotic scent. They are going from peak maturity to mature mush quickly, thus get pleasure from them whereas they last.

### INGREDIENTS

- 2 cups guava flesh
- One one/2 cups contemporary pineapple
- One banana
- 1 cup fruit crush
- One one/2 cups ice

Scoop out the complete core of the guava. To remove guava flesh, use a spoon and glide it on the guava. Blend all ingredients in till sleek.


## 13. ALMOND SMOOTHIE

The ingredients are easy-to-find, and it comes along in a real snap. It's quicker to whip this smoothie up than it has to run to the corner store for candy. Moreover, in contrast to a sweet, this smoothie can leave you feeling energized rather than groggy.

### INGREDIENTS

- ½ cup plain, sugarless almond milk
- Two tablespoons canned lightweight coconut milk

- One tablespoon sugarless chocolate
- ¾ teaspoon coconut extract
- ⅛ Teaspoon favorer
- One pinch ocean salt
- One packet stevia
- Two dates, cellular and coarsely sliced
- ½ medium banana, peeled, sliced into a pair of items, and frozen
- 2-4 ice cubes
- Two tablespoons sugarless, chopped coconut, divided

Add all ingredients into a liquidizer and method till sleek. Add the ice and pulse till mixed. Transfer to a serving glass. Stir with 1½ tablespoons chopped coconut. Sprinkle the remaining ½ tablespoon on prime and serve forthwith.


## 14. MINTY CUCUMBER WINTER MELON SMOOTHIE

I do believe that smoothies and mixed fruit and vegetable drinks are often an exquisite addition to one's diet. They're employed in moderation and with the right ingredients. Transfer a fresh, clean flavor, the mint combined with lime and sweet winter melon, to bring a reviving begin to our day.

**INGREDIENTS**

- One 1/2 Persian cucumber's, in the altogether and cut
- 1 cup cut winter melon
- 1/2 cup Greek yogurt
- Juice of one lime
- 1 tsp. torn recent mint leaves
- 2 tsp. chia seeds (optional)
- Coconut water to skinny as required

Place all ingredients into a liquidizer and puree till sleek, add many tablespoons of coconut milk if the mixture becomes too thick.


## 15. BLUEBERRY GINGER PEACH SMOOTHIE

Fresh ginger brings out the natural sweetness during this protein-packed breakfast smoothie.

**INGREDIENTS**

- One peach halved pit removed
- 1 cup blueberries
- One banana
- Two tablespoons fresh ginger
- Two scoops scoop vanilla macromolecule powder
- Two tablespoons flaxseed meal
- 1 cup of water
- Ice

Pulse all ingredients apart from the ice in an exceedingly high-speed liquidizer till sleek. Add ice till you have reached desired consistency. Serve in 2 tall glasses.

## TOP FIVE KETO RECIPES FOR HEAVY MEAL
## 1.  KETO TACOS

These cheese taco shells are perfect to start a great meal with keto. Baked cheese formed into the shape of a taco. Filled taco with seasoned ground beef for a low carb taco night.

## INGREDIENTS

- 2 cups Cheddar cheese, shredded
- 1 pound meat
- 1/4 cup Water
- 2 tablespoon Taco Sauce
- Taco is topping with Sour cream, Avocado, cheese, lettuce, etc.

## INSTRUCTION

- Preheat the oven on 350 degrees F. On a baking sheet lined with parchment paper, place 1/4 cup piles of cheese. Press the cheese down, so it makes one layer.
- Place the baking sheet in the oven — Bake for 5-7 minutes.
- Let the cheese cool for some minutes until it is firm to lift. Lift the cheese and place it over a spoon that is balanced on two cups.
- Let the cheese cool completely. Then remove the cheese.
- Place taco shells with the ground beef over medium-high heat on oven. Cook until it cooked perfectly.
- Squeeze the grease from the meat and then add the homemade taco toppings. Pour water into the skillet and stir everything around, mixing it together.

- Steam for 5 minutes.  Add meat to taco shells. Add your favorite taco toppings.

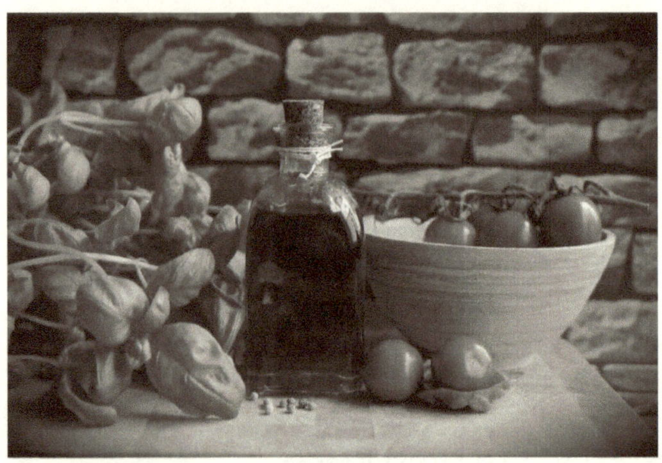

## 2.  LOADED CAULIFLOWER

This loaded cauliflower is the ultimate in low carb comfort food.

### INGREDIENTS

- 1 pound cauliflower
- 1 cup grated cheddar cheese
- Two slices cooked bacon crumbled
- Two tablespoons snipped chives
- Three tablespoons butter
- 4 ounces sour cream
- salt and pepper to taste
- 1/4 teaspoon garlic powder

### INSTRUCTIONS

- Cut the cauliflower and add them to a microwave bowl. With two tablespoons of water cover using lit. Microwave for 5-8 minutes, on your microwave, until completely cooked. Drain the water and let sit uncovered for a minute.
- Mix the butter, garlic powder, and sour cream and process until it has the required consistency. Remove the mashed cauliflower to a bowl. Add half of the cheese and mix by hand. Sprinkle salt and pepper on top.

- Top the cauliflower with the remaining cheese and bacon. Place into the microwave to melt the cheese. Then serve.

## 3. SALAD IN JAR

Pack the salad in a jar and fill with delicious salmon or chicken and dressing for a quick low-carb lunch.

### INGREDIENTS

- 1 oz. leafy greens
- ½ scallion, sliced
- One carrot
- One avocado
- 1 oz. red bell peppers
- 1 oz. cherry tomatoes
- 4 oz. smoked salmon or rotisserie chicken
- ¼ cup mayonnaise or olive oil

### INSTRUCTIONS

- Shred or chop the vegetables.
- First, put the dark leafy greens at the bottom of the jar.
- Add scallion, carrot, Avocado, bell peppers, and tomato in layers.
- Top with smoked salmon or grilled chicken.

## 4. KETO SMOKED SALMON AND AVOCADO PLATE

Real food on a plate-like Smoked salmon with Avocado. A keto dinner should be simple and easy.

### INGREDIENTS

- 7 oz. smoked salmon
- Two avocados
- ½ cup mayonnaise
- salt and pepper

### INSTRUCTIONS

- Split the Avocado in half. Scoop out avocado pieces with a spoon. Place the Avocado on the bowl.
- Add salmon and mayonnaise to the bowl with the Avocado.
- Top with freshly ground black pepper and a sprinkle of sea salt.

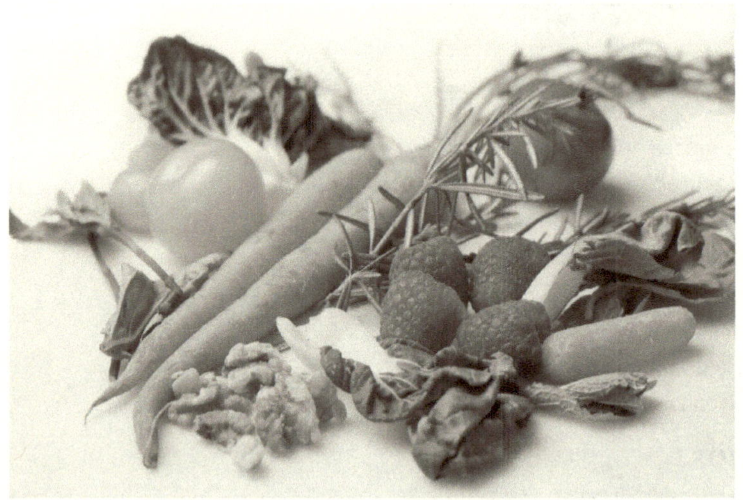

## 5.  BAKED PESTO CHICKEN

Pesto sauce is one of my favorite from all the sauces. It is perfect for quick meals. Pesto has a lot of flavor in a small package. At the end of the summer, it is perfect for a meal.

### INGREDIENTS

- 3 tbsp. basil pesto
- 1/2 tsp. salt
- 8 oz. mozzarella cheese sliced
- 1/4 tsp. black pepper for sprinkle

### INSTRUCTIONS

- Preheat oven to 350 degrees F.

- Spray baking dish with cooking oil. Place chicken in the bottom in a layer sprinkle with salt. Add some pepper to the chicken.
- Spread the pesto on the dish. Put the mozzarella cheese on the upper layer.
- Bake the dish for 35-45 minutes until the chicken cooked and the cheese melted. You can boil it for a few minutes at the end to brown the cheese if you want.

## CONCLUSION

Integrating keto recipes into your traditional diet will have tremendous health advantages. You'll be able to relish smoothies for weight loss, as a natural cleanse, to stay you hydrous, keep your bowels regular, and lots of additional advantages. Strive to experiment with totally different recipes until you discover those you actually like and can drink typically.

For effective weight loss, it's necessary to 1st eliminate these toxins through detoxification before occurring any weight loss program. Smoothies and keto recipes don't seem to be solely smart for eliminating excess toxins within the body; they additionally facilitate to heal the body and improve overall health.

In this book, you may realize an in-depth guide to assist you to come through fast and effective weight loss with keto diet through detoxification and fat loss. It might additionally teach you ways to eat healthily and train your body to begin to desire healthy foods naturally.

# END

www.ingramcontent.com/pod-product-compliance
Lightning Source LLC
Chambersburg PA
CBHW051139250726

48655CB00007B/3145